Weight loss meal prep for starters

Step by step guide in preparation of meal to achieve weight loss

Mary Hoover

Table of contents

Introduction

It's crucial to understand that your diet is crucial to attaining your goals when starting a weight-loss program. Meal planning, also referred to as "meal prep," is an effective weight loss strategy. This section of our guide's introduction will go into detail about why meal preparation is crucial for weight reduction and how setting attainable weight loss goals is the key to success.

Why Meal Planning is Important for Weight Loss

Meal planning is more than just a trendy buzzword; it's an actual, workable plan for anyone trying to lose extra weight. Here are some strong arguments for why meal planning is essential to a successful weight loss journey:

Portion Control: The ability to manage portion sizes is one of the main benefits of meal preparation for weight loss. You're less likely to overeat or give in to the lure of unhealthy snacks when you prepare your meals ahead of time. You can more easily keep to your calorie objectives by pre-portioning your food.

Balanced Nutrition: Meal prepping gives you the ability to create healthful, well-balanced meals. You may make sure that the proper ratio of proteins, carbs, and good fats is present on your plate. This well-rounded strategy supports long-term weight loss promotion, hunger reduction, and blood sugar level stabilization.

Cutting off impulse consumption of food: When we feel hungry in our busy lives, it is all very easy to get quick, routinely unhealthy meals and snacks. By making healthy selections easily available, meal preparation helps you avoid making calorie-dense, impulsive food choices.

Timing and Convenience: Meal preparation doesn't have to take a lot of time, despite what some people might think. In actuality, it can ultimately save you time. You may free up time during the hectic weekdays and lessen the stress of deciding what to eat by allocating a chunk of your week to meal planning and preparation.

Consistency is Important: Consistency is necessary for the progressive process of weight loss. Meal preparation helps you develop a habit where you consistently eat wholesome, moderately sized meals. The secret to obtaining and keeping a healthy weight is consistency.

Reduced Stress: Making the choice of what to eat each day might be stressful. By providing you with a clear strategy and ensuring you have the necessary components on hand, meal preparation reduces your stress.

Setting realistic weight loss objectives is step one.

Setting realistic weight loss goals is essential before delving into the finer points of meal preparation. Why this stage is essential to your success is as follows:

Motivation and Attention: Motivation and attention are provided by specific, attainable goals. They assist you maintain your commitment to your weight loss quest by giving you something to strive for.

Monitoring Progress: Monitoring your progress is made easier with realistic goals. Setting clear, attainable goals allows you to track your progress and make any required adjustments along the way.

Eliminating Anger: Goals that are unrealistic, like hoping for a speedy and drastic weight loss, can cause anger and disappointment. A sustained approach to weight loss is encouraged by setting attainable goals, which also minimize burnout.

Health and safety: Rapid weight reduction or extreme dieting might be harmful to your health. Realistic objectives put your health first and make sure you're losing weight in a healthy and sustainable way.

Creating Habits: Setting attainable goals gives you the chance to develop good habits. You'll develop new habits and routines that support long-term success as you work toward your goals.

Meal planning is a crucial weight loss approach that provides advantages including portion control, balanced nutrition, and stress reduction. It's important to start your journey with attainable weight loss objectives, though. These objectives act as a guide to help you go where you want to go, keeping you motivated and secure as you go. As we move deeper into this guide, you'll learn useful advice and tactics to help you make the most of meal planning and reach your weight reduction objectives.

Understanding the Foundations of Nutrition

It's imperative to understand the basics of nutrition before starting your weight loss journey through meal preparation. This information will help you decide what to put in your meals and how to balance them for successful weight loss. The role of calories in weight loss and the significance of maintaining a balance among macronutrients—namely, protein, carbs, and fats—will both be covered in this section.

Calorie Intake and Weight Loss

Your body uses calories as the basic unit of energy for all of its processes, including breathing and physical activity. You must consume less calories than your body uses in order to develop a calorie deficit and lose weight. Here are some reasons why it's critical for you to comprehend how calories affect weight loss:

Caloric Balance: You must consume less calories each day than you expend in order to lose weight. By causing a deficit, this forces your body to burn stored fat for energy, which causes weight loss.

Long-Term Weight Loss: For long-lasting weight loss, a moderate calorie deficit is essential. Extreme calorie restriction can result in unsustainable diets, muscle loss, and vitamin deficiencies. You can achieve the appropriate balance by being aware of your daily caloric requirements.

Monitoring Progress: You can successfully track your progress by keeping an eye on your caloric intake. It gives you a clear view of your progress toward your weight loss objectives.

Mindful Eating: Mindful eating is encouraged by calorie awareness. You become more aware of the foods you eat and how they affect the number of calories you consume each day.

A customized strategy to weight loss is possible when you are aware of your particular calorie requirements. Your daily calorie needs depend on things like your age, gender, degree of activity, and metabolism.

Achieving Macronutrient Balance with Protein, Carbs, and Fats

It's critical to pay attention to the macronutrients you consume, which are protein, carbs, and fats, in addition to controlling your calorie consumption. Your ability to successfully lose weight depends on how well you balance these macronutrients:

Protein: Your body is made up primarily of proteins. It is necessary for feeling full and pleased and helps with muscle growth and repair. Lean protein foods, such chicken, fish, tofu, and beans, can help you maintain muscle mass while shedding fat.

Carbohydrates: Energy-producing carbohydrates are essential to a balanced diet. Choose complex carbohydrates instead, such as whole grains, fruits, and vegetables, as they offer satiating, long-lasting energy and fiber.

Fats: Several biological processes, including hormone production and nutrient absorption, depend on healthy fats. Limit saturated and trans fats in your diet while increasing sources of unsaturated fats like avocados, almonds, and olive oil.

Portion Control: Portion control is a necessary component in balancing macronutrients. Portion control is important since consuming too much of any macronutrient can result in weight gain. Utilize meal preparation to make well-balanced meals and manage portion sizes.

Individual Needs: Depending on your activity level, age, and health objectives, your macronutrient requirements could change. Finding your appropriate macronutrient ratio can be done with the aid of internet calculators or by seeing a nutritionist.

In conclusion, the fundamentals of nutrition and weight loss are an awareness of the function of calories and maintaining a balance of macronutrients. You create a strong basis for your food preparation efforts by learning these fundamentals. In the parts that follow, we'll look at how to put this information into practice to cook scrumptious meals that are healthy and supportive of your weight loss objectives.

Chapter 1

Kitchen necessities

Having the proper equipment and supplies on hand is essential if you want to start a successful weight loss program involving meal preparation. The essential kitchen utensils and how to stock a wholesome pantry are the two key topics covered in this section of the guide.

Essential Kitchen Tools

The appropriate kitchenware may improve the efficiency and enjoyment of meal preparation. Here is a list of essential kitchen appliances for efficient meal preparation for weight loss:

Cutting board and good knives: To chop fruits, veggies, and proteins effectively and safely, you'll need a solid cutting board and sharp blades.

Measurement cups and spoons: The key to weight loss is precise portion control, which measuring cups and spoons help you do.

The food scale When weighing ingredients, a digital food scale is essential for accurate calorie and macronutrient calculations.

Pots & Pans: For cooking a variety of dishes, from stir-fries to soups, a set of high-quality pots and pans with non-stick surfaces is required.

Ovenware and baking sheets: These are essential for baking and roasting foods like lean proteins or vegetables on a sheet pan.

Food processor or blender: These kitchen tools can be used to make sauces, purees, and smoothies.

Instant Pot or Slow Cooker: These appliances make cooking convenient and can be used to quickly prepare nutritious meals that are cooked slowly.

Meal preparation containers: Purchase a range of meal prep containers in various sizes to portion and safely store your prepared meals.

A kitchen thermometer makes sure that your proteins are prepared to the proper internal temperature for food safety.

Grater and Zester are: With components like cheese, citrus zest, and spices, you can easily add flavor and texture to your recipes with the help of these instruments.

Salad Spinner: Use it to quickly wash and dry leafy greens and herbs.

Tongs and spatulas: These can be used in a variety of ways to flip, toss, and serve food without hurting it.

Microwave: Effective for swiftly reheating prepared meals.

Cutting Shears These scissors work well for cutting plants and unwrapping food containers.

Peeler: Beneficial for peeling fruits and vegetables.

Building a Healthy Pantry

A well-stocked pantry is essential for effective meal preparation. To prepare a nutritious pantry for your weight reduction endeavor, follow these steps:

Whole Grains: Include options for fiber-rich, satisfying carbohydrates such brown rice, quinoa, whole wheat pasta, and oats.

Canned goods: For simple additions to meals, choose low-sodium canned beans, tomatoes, and veggies.

Healthy Oils: For frying and dressing, pick coconut, avocado, or olive oil.

Build a collection of herbs and spices to flavor your food without adding too many calories.

Lean Proteins: Purchase plenty of tuna, salmon, and lean turkey or chicken in cans. Think about tempeh and tofu for plant-based protein.

Nuts and seeds:For healthy fats and protein, add almonds, walnuts, chia seeds, and flaxseeds.

Nut Butter: Choose organic nut butters free of hydrogenated oils or additional sweeteners.

Boiling water and Bouillons: When preparing soups and meals, pick low-sodium options.

Keep staple condiments like mustard, spicy sauce, vinegar, and low-sugar ketchup on hand for flavor.

The sweeteners are: Use substitutes for sugar, such as honey, maple syrup, or stevia.

Dried Fruits: These can naturally sweeten foods if used sparingly.

Choose canned fruits that are in their juices or water rather than those that are packed in thick syrups.

Whole-grain flour: Consider using whole wheat or almond flour if you like to bake.

You'll be prepared for successful meal preparation for weight loss if you have these cooking tools and a fully stocked pantry. In the parts that follow, we'll delve into using these components to make wholesome and delectable meals.

Chapter 2

Meal preparation

A key element of effective weight loss through meal preparation is meal planning. It enables you to take charge of your nutrition, make wise food decisions, and make sure that you are achieving your nutritional objectives. The creation of a weekly meal plan and mastering portion control and serving sizes are the two key components of meal planning that will be covered in this section.

Making a Weekly Meal Plan

Setting up a weekly meal plan is similar to plotting your course for weight loss. It gives you guidelines, stops irrational eating, and gives you variety of options to select from. Here is a step-by-step tutorial for making a successful meal plan:

Establish your weight loss objectives and food preferences first (point a). Are you looking for precise macronutrient ratios or a set daily calorie intake? Do you have any dietary preferences or limits, such as being vegetarian or gluten-free? This will give you guide in planning your meal

b. Arrange Your Meals: Eat three meals and one or two snacks throughout the day, usually breakfast, lunch, and dinner. Give each meal a specific objective: breakfast for vigor, lunch for nourishment, and dinner for a well-rounded day's end.

Choose foods that are nutrient-dense: Concentrate on including nutrient-dense items in your diet, such as fruits, vegetables, lean proteins, whole grains, and healthy fats. These meals supply important vitamins and minerals without having too many calories.

Variety is Important: To avoid being bored and to make sure you're getting a variety of nutrients, plan for variety in your meals. Throughout the week, switch up your proteins, vegetables, and grains.

Prepare beforehand: Choose foods that can be prepared in advance and cooked in bulk. Take into account dishes that may be portioned out for numerous meals and cooked in larger quantities.

Plan for occasional treats or indulgences while staying inside your calorie budget. The hidden fact to success at the long-run is moderation

Be Practical: When making meal plans, take your schedule into account. Make sure your strategy allows for simple execution and fits with your daily schedule.

Make a shopping list: Make a shopping list with all the ingredients you'll need after you've decided on your menu. By doing this, you may reduce food waste and make sure you have everything.

Tracking Progress: Use a food journal or a meal monitoring app to document your intake as you stick to your meal plan. This will make you to be accountable and make changes where necessary

serving sizes, and portion control

Meal planning must include serving sizes and portion control, especially if weight loss is the goal. Here's why they're important:

Calorie Control: You may prevent accidentally consuming too many calories by controlling your portions properly. If eaten in big numbers, even nutritious meals can cause weight gain.

Mindful Eating: Mindful eating is encouraged by portion control. It enables you to enjoy your meals, determine when you are full, and avoid overeating.

Balanced Meals: By managing portion proportions, you can prepare healthy meals that support your nutritional objectives. Each meal can contain the ideal proportion of protein, carbs, and fats.

As you are less likely to prepare or order more food than you can properly consume, portion management helps to decrease food waste.

Visual Supports Learn how to recognize portion sizes visually. For instance, a meal of lean protein is approximately the size of your palm, a serving of carbohydrates is around the size of your cupped hand, and a serving of healthy fats is about the size of your thumb.

Use meal preparation containers: To make it simple to store and transport your prepared meals without overeating, invest in portion-controlled meal prep containers.

Exercise Moderation: Keep in mind that eating your favorite meals while exercising portion control is still acceptable. Finding a balance and including treats into your overall calorie goals are key.

You'll be well-equipped to successfully traverse your weight reduction journey if you develop a weekly food plan and become an expert at portion control. These routines give you direction, encourage mindful eating, and make sure you're taking care of your body while pursuing your objectives. In the sections that follow, we'll look at useful meal preparation techniques and dishes to make your plan a reality.

Chapter 3

Shopping for groceries

A vital part of keeping a balanced diet and reaching your weight loss objectives is grocery shopping. You should concentrate on creating a healthy food list and using smart shopping techniques to get the most out of your supermarket outings. Both of these crucial components will be covered in detail in this section.

Creating a List of Healthful Groceries

A successful weight reduction and meal preparation journey is built on a well-planned grocery list. Here's how to create a list of healthful foods to buy:

Meal preparation: Plan out your meals for the week before you go shopping. Describe the meals you'll be making for breakfast, lunch, dinner, and snacks. Your shopping list will be guided by this.

Give fresh produce top priority: List a range of fresh fruits and veggies to start. To make sure you're getting a variety of vitamins and minerals, aim for a rainbow of colors.

Lean Proteins: Include lean protein sources in your list. Skinless chicken, lean beef or pig, fish, tofu, beans, lentils, and low-fat dairy products are examples of this.

Include whole grains such as brown rice, quinoa, whole wheat pasta, oats, and whole-grain bread in your diet. These offer necessary fiber and ongoing energy.

Healthy Fats: Olive oil, almonds, seeds, and avocados are just a few examples of sources of healthful fats. These are critical for satiety and general health.

Dairy products or dairy substitutes: If you consume dairy products, think about low-fat or Greek yogurt, skim milk, and low-fat cheese. If you prefer plant-based alternatives or are lactose intolerant, choose unsweetened dairy substitutes like almond or soy milk.

Treats and Snacks: Greek yogurt, diced veggies, fresh fruit, or unsalted nuts are all good options for healthful snacking. Occasionally include goodies, but pay attention to portion amounts.

Foods that are frozen and canned: Stock up on frozen fruits and veggies, canned tomatoes, and canned beans. These are more readily available and last longer.

Spices and herbs: Spice up your food with herbs and spices. Think about basic ingredients like cumin, cinnamon, oregano, basil, and garlic.

Condiments To improve the flavor of your food, use condiments like mustard, spicy sauce, vinegar, and low-sugar ketchup.

Beverages: Drink plenty of fluids and think about low-calorie options like sparkling water or unsweetened tea.

Review Labels: Read labels thoroughly before purchasing packaged items. Look for products with little to no added sodium, sugar, or bad fats.

Plan Ahead for Leftovers: Plan one or more meals based on the leftovers from earlier meals. This saves time and lessens food waste.

Fresh Goods Shopping: Visit the store at the conclusion of your vacation to buy perishable things like dairy and fresh produce to keep them fresh.

Smart Shopping Techniques

Making a list of healthy foods to buy is just the beginning; using smart shopping techniques can also help you save money and make healthier decisions:

Stick to a List: Refrain from making impulsive purchases by following your list. Pre-plan your meals and only purchase what you require.

Shop the Periphery: The perimeter of the store is frequently where you'll find dairy goods, fresh veggies, and lean proteins. Increase your time spent there.

Avoid Temptation-Filled Aisles: If they're not on your list, avoid the snack, sugary drink, and processed food aisles.

Buy in Bulk (for Non-Perishables): To save money in the long run, think about buying non-perishable items in bulk.

Always Read Labels: Nutritional information, component lists, and serving sizes can all be found on product labels. Choose products with less sodium, added sugar, and bad fats.

Use sales, coupons, and shop loyalty programs to save money on healthful products. Use Coupons and Discounts.

Don't Shop While Hungry: Eating something beforehand can prevent you from buying unhealthy snacks or from overspending in general.

Compare pricing: To get the most for your money, compare unit pricing (price per ounce or gram).

Select Seasonal Produce: Fruits and vegetables that are in season are sometimes cheaper and fresher. They can also provide your meals with more variety.

Verify Expiration Dates: Make sure the products you buy have a decent shelf life and are not about to expire.

Think About Frozen Produce: A quick and wholesome alternative, frozen fruits and vegetables frequently have less additives than canned counterparts.

Building a healthy grocery list and using shrewd purchasing techniques will help you succeed in your efforts to prepare healthy meals and lose weight. These techniques assist you in making sensible decisions, staying within your means, and maintaining a healthy, balanced diet.

Chapter 4

Ingredients preparation

Proper ingredient preparation is the first step in efficient meal preparation. This step guarantees that your meals are nutritional and safe in addition to being delicious. This section will examine several aspects of ingredient preparation, such as selecting lean protein sources, cleaning and chopping produce, and adding whole grains.

Washing and preparing produce correctly

The foundation of a healthy diet is a variety of fresh fruits and vegetables. Produce must be cleaned and prepared properly to assure their safety and best flavor:

Washing: All fresh produce should be given a thorough rinse in cold running water. For products like cucumbers with hard skins, use a gentle brush. Wash the produce first, even if you want to peel it, to stop any contaminates from spreading to the flesh when you cut them.

Leafy Greens: Leafy greens, such as lettuce and spinach, should be properly rinsed after being submerged in a bowl of cold water and tossed around. To get rid of extra moisture, spin salads.

Soaking: To help eliminate pesticides or bacteria, some fruits and vegetables, especially berries, benefit from a quick soak in a solution of water and vinegar (3:1 ratio). After rightly soaked, wash them thoroughly.

Preparation: Slice or chop your produce after cleaning it in accordance with your meal plan. To keep prepared fruits and vegetables fresh throughout the week, put them in airtight containers or resealable bags.

Prevent Overpreparation: Despite the convenience of prepping ahead of time, avoid chopping fruits or vegetables too much in advance because they will eventually lose their freshness and nutritional value.

Selecting Lean Protein Sources

Protein is crucial for preserving muscle mass and encouraging satiety. A healthy meal preparation starts with choosing lean protein sources:

Poultry: Turkey breast and skinless chicken are both great options. To keep them slim, trim any visible fat.

Fish: Choose lean alternatives like cod or tilapia over fatty fish like salmon, mackerel, and trout for their omega-3 fatty acids.

Lean Meat Cuts: Choose "loin" or "round"-style cuts of beef or pig since they are often thinner. Before cooking, remove any visible fat.

Tofu, tempeh, legumes (beans, lentils, and chickpeas), and quinoa are all top-notch plant-based protein sources.

Dairy products: Greek yogurt, low-fat cheese, and skim milk are examples of dairy products that are high in protein yet low in saturated fat.

Eggs: Eggs are a flexible source of protein. To lower calorie and cholesterol intake, choose egg whites or a mixture of whole eggs and egg whites.

Portion control: Pay attention to portion sizes to prevent consuming too many calories. Protein portions are around the size of your palm.

Including whole grains: Whole grains are essential to a healthy diet since they are high in fiber and minerals. Think about the following while preparing meals with whole grains:

Variety: To spice up your meals, choose a range of nutritious grains. Brown rice, quinoa, whole wheat pasta, bulgur, barley, and oats are among the choices.

Cooking Methods: To guarantee that whole grains are cooked to perfection, carefully follow the cooking guidelines. Grain can turn mushy if it is overcooked.

Batch cooking: Whole grains can be prepared in bigger batches and kept in the freezer or refrigerator for use in different meals throughout the week.

Meal Balancing: Include whole grains as a source of carbs in your meal plan to provide you long-lasting energy.

Fiber Content: **e. Whole grains contain fiber, which helps with digestion and may make you feel fuller for longer, lowering the temptation to overeat.

Portion Control: Be aware of your portion sizes because, despite being healthful, whole grains still add calories to your meals.

You may create nourishing and delectable meals by properly cleaning and preparing veggies, selecting lean protein sources, and combining whole grains. These measures make sure your ingredients are secure, savory, and in line with your dietary and health objectives.

Chapter 5

Cooking techniques

In order to prepare delicious, nutrient-dense, and weight loss-friendly meals, you must become an expert cook. This section will look at several areas of cooking, such as healthy cooking practices and ways to cut back on added sugars and fats.

Healthful cooking techniques

The nutritional value of your meals can be dramatically impacted by selecting the correct cooking techniques. Here are some healthy cooking techniques to take into account:

Grilling: Lean meats, fish, and vegetables cook beautifully on the grill. Without adding extra calories, it adds a smoky flavor. For more flavor, marinate your proteins with herbs and spices.

Baking and roasting: Vegetables and meats can be prepared in a variety of ways, including baking and roasting. To avoid sticking, use a small amount of healthy oil or cooking spray. For flavor, season with herbs and spices.

Steaming:
The nutrients in your food are retained when you steam it, a moderate cooking technique. For steaming veggies, seafood, or even grains like quinoa, use a steamer basket or a microwave-safe container with a lid.

Cooking in a skillet or stir-frying: Little oil is used in sautéing and stir-frying, making them healthier options. Lean proteins and colorful veggies should be consumed in large quantities while a nonstick skillet and little oil are used.

Poaching:Food is poached by cooking it in a flavorful liquid, most frequently water or broth. It's a great way to prepare eggs, fish, or fowl. Spice up the poaching liquor with aromatics, citrus, or herbs.

,,Cooking Slowly Hearty, low-fat meals can be easily made in a slow cooker with little effort. It works well on lean meat cuts, soups, and stews.

Steaming in Packets:Wrapping items in foil or parchment paper, steaming or baking them will create packets of ingredients. With this technique, tastes and nutrients remain contained.

h. Panini pressing or griddling: By using these techniques, you may cook without using additional oil while giving your sandwiches and proteins a great sear.

Microwave:Microwaving can be a practical technique to cook vegetables or reheat prepared meals, while being frequently disregarded for meal preparation. To ensure consistent cooking, use microwave-safe containers and adhere to the instructions.

j. Raw Material Preparation: For extra texture and nutrition, think about include raw foods like fruits, veggies, and nuts in your meals. Sushi, salads, and smoothie bowls are a few examples of raw foods.

Measurement Control: Regardless of the cooking technique you select, be mindful of portion sizes to prevent overeating and make sure your meals meet your calorie objectives.

Cutting back on added sugars and fats

In order to lose weight and improve your general health, you must cut back on additional sweets and fats in your meals. Here's an efficient way to go about it:

a. Read the labels: Learn how to read food labels to find out where packaged foods get their sources of harmful fats and added sugars. Look for products with few trans fats and extra sugars.

b. Natural Sweeteners: When necessary, use moderate amounts of natural sweeteners like honey, maple syrup, or agave nectar. Pay attention to portion sizes.

c. Limit processed food intake: Processed foods frequently have unhealthy fats and sugars hiding in them. Reduce your intake of fried foods, pre-packaged snacks, and sugary cereals.

d. Prepare food from scratch: The ingredients are under your control when you make meals from scratch. You may limit added sugars, switch to healthier cooking oils, and stay away from processed additives.

e. To add flavor, use herbs and spices: To boost flavor without adding calories, swap salt and sugar with herbs, spices, and other seasonings.

f. Use wholesome fats: For their heart-healthy fats, choose cooking oils like olive oil, avocado oil, or coconut oil. To limit overall calorie intake, use them sparingly.

g. Pay Attention to Portion Sizes Even natural carbohydrates and good fats can cause weight gain if ingested in excess. When using these ingredients, pay attention to serving sizes.

h. Try Different Cooking Methods: To lower your overall fat intake, experiment with different cooking methods that don't rely on extra fats, such baking, grilling, and steaming.

i. Dairy Alternatives: When preparing or cooking foods with dairy ingredients, choose low-fat or reduced-fat dairy products.

j. Prevent Drinks With Sugar:** A large source of added sugars can come from sugary drinks like soda and sweetened fruit juices. Instead, choose unsweetened beverages, water, or herbal tea.

You may prepare tasty, nutritious meals that help your weight loss objectives by using smart cooking techniques and being aware of additional sugars and fats. These methods enable you to partake in gratifying meals without sacrificing flavor

Chapter 6

Breakfast suggestion

Breakfast is frequently regarded as the most crucial meal of the day, and it can have a big impact on your efforts to lose weight. This section will discuss many breakfast options, such as nutrient-dense breakfast meals and quick and simple morning options.

Recipes for nutrient-rich breakfasts

A nutrient-rich breakfast helps to nourish your body throughout the morning and sets a good mood for the rest of the day. Here are a few tempting and healthy breakfast recipes to take into account:

Oats overnight: Rollin oats should be combined with Greek yogurt, milk or a milk substitute, and any desired garnishes, such as fresh fruit, nuts, seeds, or a drizzle of honey. For a quick, no-cook breakfast, place it in the refrigerator overnight.

Vegetable Omelet: Toss eggs or egg whites with diced spinach, tomatoes, onions, and bell peppers. For a breakfast that is loaded with vegetables and protein, cook in a nonstick skillet with a little olive oil.

Greek yogurt parfait: For a creamy and filling breakfast, top Greek yogurt with oats, fruit, and a dash of almonds.

Avocado Toast: For a nutrient-dense and satisfying dinner, spread mashed avocado on whole-grain toast and top with sliced tomatoes, a poached egg, and a dash of salt and pepper.

Smoothie Bowl: Make a thick, creamy smoothie by blending your favorite fruits, veggies, Greek yogurt, and one scoop of protein powder (if preferred). For extra texture and nutrients, sprinkle on some granola, nuts, and fruit slices.

Chia Seed Pudding: Chia seeds should be combined with milk (or a milk substitute), sugar, and vanilla essence. For a meal that is high in fiber and protein, let it sit in the refrigerator overnight. The next morning, top with fresh fruit and a few chopped almonds.

Pancakes made with whole grains: To add more fiber to your pancakes, use whole wheat or oat flour. Greek yogurt, fresh berries, and a drizzle of pure maple syrup should be added on top.

Breakfast Burrito: For a flavorful, protein-rich breakfast, pile scrambled eggs, black beans, sautéed spinach, and salsa inside a whole-wheat tortilla.

Quinoa Breakfast Bowl (i) Cook quinoa with milk or a milk substitute and add honey or maple syrup for sweetness. For a breakfast strong in protein and made with grains, top with almonds, dried fruit, and a dollop of Greek yogurt.

Bowl of cottage cheese: For a protein-rich and filling breakfast, combine cottage cheese with sliced fruits (such as peaches or pineapple), a drizzle of honey, and a sprinkling of cinnamon.

 Quick and simple breakfast options

Even though mornings can be busy, you shouldn't forgo a filling meal. Following are some quick and simple breakfast ideas for hectic mornings:

Toast with peanut butter and bananas: On a slice of whole grain toast, spread peanut butter. Add banana slices and finish with chia seeds or honey.

Fruit and Nut Butter Wrap: For a portable breakfast, spread almond or peanut butter on a whole-grain tortilla, top with strawberry or apple slices, and roll it up.

High-Fiber Cereal: Pick a cereal high in fiber, such as bran flakes or shredded wheat, and add skim milk or a milk substitute on top.

Shake with protein: For a quick and nutrient-rich breakfast on the go, blend a scoop of protein powder with water or milk, a handful of spinach, and a frozen banana.

Grab-and-Go Yogurt: For a quick and easy breakfast, grab a single-serving container of Greek yogurt and some fruit before you leave the house.

Hard-boiled eggs: For a portable, high-protein breakfast, hard boil eggs in advance. Add some fruit or whole-grain crackers to go with them.

Trail Mix: For a fast and energizing breakfast, mix nuts, seeds, and dried fruits to make your own trail mix.

Remainings: Feel free to eat the supper leftovers from last night for breakfast. A grilled chicken breast or some roasted veggies can be healthy options.

Whole Fruit: As you leave the house, grab a piece of whole fruit, like an apple or a banana. To increase satiety, serve it with a tiny handful of nuts.

These breakfast suggestions provide you a variety of options, from nutrient-dense dishes to quick and simple selections, so you may choose breakfasts that suit your schedule and preferences. You may put yourself on the road to success in your weight loss goal by beginning the day with a balanced and nourishing breakfast.

Chapter 7

Recipes for lunch

Lunch is a crucial component of your daily diet and can have a big impact on your attempts to lose weight. We'll look at a variety of lunch meals in this area, including full and well-balanced lunch options as well as straightforward and wholesome salad recipes.

Ideas for Filling and Balanced Lunches

You may stay motivated and satisfied throughout the rest of the day with a balanced and substantial lunch. Here are some scrumptious and healthy lunch ideas to think about:

Wrap with grilled chicken and vegetables: Grilled chicken breast, mixed greens, roasted veggies, and a mild dressing should all be placed inside a whole-grain wrap. For a filling and portable lunch, roll it up.

Salad of quinoa and black beans:Black beans, corn, cherry tomatoes, red onion, and cilantro should be combined with cooked quinoa. Add a lime vinaigrette for a delicious and protein-rich salad.

Lettuce wraps with turkey and avocado (optional) Wrap lean turkey slices, avocado, tomato, and a dollop of Greek yogurt or hummus inside of large lettuce leaves.

Lentil and Veggie Soup:Use low-sodium broth, lots of vegetables, and cooked lentils to make a substantial lentil and vegetable soup. For flavor, season with herbs and spices.

Greek yogurt and tuna salad:Greek yogurt, sliced celery, red onion, and a squeeze of lemon juice are combined with canned tuna. Serve with whole wheat toast or whole grain crackers.

Quinoa and Chickpea Bowl:Put cooked quinoa, chickpeas, cucumber, bell pepper, and feta cheese in a bowl. For a dish with a Mediterranean flair, drizzle with olive oil and lemon juice.

Turkey and vegetable stir-fry: Sauté a variety of bright veggies, including bell peppers, broccoli, and snap peas, with lean ground turkey. Serve over brown rice or cauliflower rice and season with low-sodium soy sauce.

Whole-Wheat Pasta Salad: Use whole grain spaghetti, cherry tomatoes, cucumbers, olives, and feta cheese to make a pasta salad. Dress with fresh basil and balsamic vinaigrette.

Burrito Bowl with Beans and Veggies: Brown rice that has been cooked is layered with black beans, peppers and onions that have been sautéed, shredded lettuce, chopped tomatoes, and a dollop of guacamole or Greek yogurt.

Chicken Breast Stuffed with Spinach and Feta:Chicken breast should be stuffed with spinach and feta cheese before being baked till done. Green beans or broccoli on the side, steamed.

Salad of sweet potatoes and black beans: For a tasty and substantial salad, roast sweet potato cubes and combine them with black beans, corn, red onion, and a honey-lime dressing.

Wrap with vegetables and hummus: On a whole-grain wrap, spread hummus and top with carrot sticks, thinly sliced cucumber, bell pepper, and mixed greens. For a cool and filling lunch, roll it up.

Quick and Healthy Salad Recipes

Because of their adaptability, salads can be a go-to lunch choice. Here are a few quick and wholesome salad recipes to try:

The traditional Cobb salad Grilled chicken, hard-boiled eggs, avocado, cherry tomatoes, and crumbled bacon should all be added to mixed greens. Apply a thin vinaigrette to the dish.
Greek Salad:Combine cucumbers, feta cheese, Kalamata olives, cherry tomatoes, red onion, and Greek dressing. Serve with some pita bread that has been grilled.

Caprese salad Place tomato, basil, and fresh mozzarella slices on a platter. In addition, put pepper and salt then drizzle with balsamic glaze.

Asian-influenced salad: Combine cooked and cooled rice noodles with chopped cabbage, carrots, and cucumber. Add grilled tofu or shrimp on top, along with a sesame ginger dressing.

Berry and spinach salad, e.g. Baby spinach it should be combined with goat cheese, candied walnuts, and fresh berries. Use a balsamic vinaigrette to dress.

Salad of quinoa and kale: Combine cooked quinoa with diced red bell pepper, chopped kale, dried cranberries, and goat cheese. Add a lemon-tahini dressing and toss.

Taco Salad:Crushed tortilla chips, cooked mince beef or turkey, black beans, chopped tomatoes, and mixed greens are layered on top. Add Greek yogurt and salsa to the top.

Grilled chicken Caesar salad Grilled chicken breast, whole-grain croutons, and a light Caesar dressing are combined with romaine lettuce in a salad. Add some Parmesan cheese.

Chickpea salad from the Mediterranean: Combine sliced cucumber, cherry tomatoes, red onion, parsley, and feta cheese with the chickpeas. Dress with a dressing of lemon and olive oil.

Waldorf Salad:Greek yogurt, a little honey, and sliced apples, celery, grapes, and walnuts are combined. On a bed of mixed greens, serve.

Chapter 8

Recipes for dinner

The opportunity to eat a filling, healthy, and balanced meal is presented by dinner, which is frequently the last meal of the day. We'll look at a range of dinner recipes in this area, including nutritious options, one-pot meals, and stir-fry dishes.

Healthy Dinner Options

By offering vital nutrition and satisfaction, a filling meal can help you finish the day strong. Here are some scrumptious and healthy dinner recipes to take into account:

Salmon on the grill with quinoa and asparagus in a steaming broth: Salmon filets grilled with lemon and herbs seasoning. For a well-rounded supper, serve with cooked quinoa and steamed asparagus.

Bell Peppers Stuffed: Diced tomatoes, brown rice, lean ground turkey, and spices are combined and put inside bell peppers. Add cheese on top after baking the dish until it is soft.

Chili that is vegetarian:Beans (pinto, kidney, and black beans), diced tomatoes, onions, and a variety of spices are used to make a robust chili. Serve alongside whole-grain cornbread or rice.

Roasted vegetables and baked chicken: Roasted carrots, broccoli, and red potatoes are served with boneless, skinless chicken breasts that have been spiced.

Spaghetti Squash with Turkey Meatballs and Tomato Sauce: Serving suggestions: Roast spaghetti squash, shred it into "noodles," top with homemade tomato sauce and lean turkey meatballs.

Curry made with lentils and vegetables: Lentils, diced tomatoes, onions, and an assortment of Indian spices are used to make a vegetable curry. Over brown rice, please.

Broccoli and Tofu Stir-Fried: Broccoli florets and tofu cubes are sautéed in a sesame ginger stir-fry sauce. Serve with whole wheat noodles or brown rice.

Sweet potato and black bean quesadillas baked in the oven: Sweet potato mash, black beans, and shredded cheese are layered between whole-grain tortillas to create quesadillas. till crispy, bake.

Quinoa-topped grilled shrimp dish with sautéed spinach: Garlic and herbs are used for grilling shrimp. Serve with quinoa and spinach that has been sautéed in oil.

The Ratatouille movie: With eggplant, zucchini, bell peppers, tomatoes, and onions cooked in a tomato sauce, make a vibrant ratatouille. Serve alongside whole-grain couscous or on top of it.

Zoodles with pesto served with grilled chicken: For a low-carb dinner option, spiralize zucchini to make "zoodles," combine with homemade pesto, and top with grilled chicken.

Salmon with Teriyaki Glaze, Steamed Broccoli, and Brown Rice: For a healthy Asian-inspired lunch, prepare fish with a teriyaki sauce and serve it with steamed broccoli and brown rice.

Recipes for one-pot meals and stir-fries

Stir-fry dishes and one-pot dinners are not only practical but also flavorful and nutrient-dense. Try some of these:

Stir-fry with chicken and vegetables: In a light stir-fry sauce consisting of low-sodium soy sauce, ginger, and garlic, sauté chicken

breast pieces with a variety of vibrant veggies. Serve with quinoa or brown rice.
Stir-fry with beef and broccoli: Lean beef that has been thinly sliced is stir-fried with broccoli, ginger, and a flavorful sauce. Serve with noodles or rice.

Vegetable and Chickpea Curry in One Pot: Cook canned tomatoes, chickpeas, and various veggies in a tasty curry sauce made with coconut milk and spices.

White bean and sausage stew: Lean turkey or chicken sausage, white beans, kale, and a tomato-based broth can all be combined to create a substantial stew.

Stir-fry with shrimp and vegetables: Shrimp should be stir-fried quickly with bell peppers of various colors, snap peas, and a ginger-soy sauce. Serve with whole wheat noodles or brown rice.

Rice and Chicken in One Pot: For a quick, tasty lunch, sauté chicken pieces, onions, and bell peppers before simmering with brown rice, diced tomatoes, and seasonings in a single pot.
It
Stir-Fry with Spicy Thai Noodles Cook rice noodles and combine them with bean sprouts, shredded carrots, sautéed tofu or shrimp, and a hot Thai peanut sauce.

Quinoa and vegetable pilaf made in one pot: For a filling one-pot meal, sauté a variety of veggies, including carrots, peas, and bell peppers, before adding quinoa and vegetable broth.

Pad Thai with vegetables and tofu: Combine soy sauce, lime juice, and peanut butter to make a homemade pad Thai sauce, then stir-fry tofu and a variety of vegetables. Add rice noodles and sprinkle chopped peanuts over top.

Skillet with Italian sausage and vegetables: Sauté onions, zucchini, and colorful bell peppers with Italian sausage. Spices and canned tomatoes can be added to a skillet meal to add flavor.

These supper recipes provide a variety of options, including healthy selections, one-pot meals, and stir-fry dishes. You may maintain a healthy eating habit and assist your weight loss objectives by preparing balanced and filling dinners.

Side dishes and Snacks

Your total diet and weight loss efforts may be significantly impacted by your choice of snacks and sides. They offer chances to savor a range of flavors and nutrients all day long. We'll discuss wholesome snack options and delectable side dishes to go with your meals in this section.

Healthy Snack Options,

Between-meal satisfaction can be achieved with nutritious snacks that also supply necessary nutrients. Here are some options for healthy and satiating snacks:

Greek yogurt with fruit Greek yogurt has a lot of calcium and protein. For a delightful and powerful source of antioxidants, top it with fresh berries.

Hummus and vegetables: Enjoy a serving of hummus with sliced cucumbers, bell peppers, or baby carrots for a filling and crispy snack.

Apples dipped in nut butter: For a sweet and protein-rich snack, slice apples and mix them with almond, peanut, or cashew butter.

Mixed Nuts:A little handful of unsalted mixed nuts can give you a delightful crunch, good fats, and protein.

Pineapple and cottage cheese: For a protein-rich and sweet snack, combine low-fat cottage cheese with fresh pineapple chunks.

Hard-boiled eggs (f) Hard-boiled eggs can be made ahead of time and eaten as a portable, protein-rich snack.

Trail Mix:For a balanced snack, mix nuts, seeds, dried fruits, and a little dark chocolate to make your own trail mix.

Avocado and Rice Cakes: For a filling and creamy snack, spread mashed avocado on whole-grain rice cakes and season with a dash of salt and pepper.

"Edamame" For a healthy and protein-rich snack, lightly season steamed edamame (young soybeans) with sea salt.

Popcorn: For a whole-grain, high-fiber snack, air-pop or briefly microwave popcorn. For a cheesy flavor, season with a light sprinkle of nutritional yeast.

Vegetable Chips: By thinly slicing sweet potatoes, zucchini, or beets and baking them until crisp, you can make your own vegetable chips.

Chia Pudding Almond milk, chia seeds, and a little honey should be combined. For a snack high in fiber, let it sit in the refrigerator until it thickens.

Banana slices with peanut butter: piece a banana and spread peanut butter on each piece for a pleasant and energy-boosting snack.

Roasted Chickpeas:For a protein-rich, delicious snack, season chickpeas with your preferred spices and roast them until crunchy.

Guacamole-topped veggie sticks Dip celery, carrot, and cucumber sticks into homemade or store-bought guacamole for a creamy and nutrient-rich snack.

Mini Caprese Skewers:On toothpicks, arrange cherry tomatoes, fresh basil leaves, and tiny mozzarella balls. Balsamic glaze can be drizzled for a tasty snack.

Chapter 9

Delicious side dishes

Your major meals can be complemented by side dishes, which can also diversify your diet. Here are some delectable suggestions for sides:

Roasted vegetables include: For a tasty side, roast a variety of seasonal veggies with olive oil and your preferred seasonings.

Quinoa Salad: Toss cooked quinoa with chopped cucumber, bell peppers, cherry tomatoes, fresh herbs, and a lemon vinaigrette.

Garlic Mashed Cauliflower:Steam cauliflower and mash it with roasted garlic, a touch of butter or olive oil, and low-fat milk for a creamy side.

Sautéed Spinach with Garlic:For a quick and wholesome side dish, quickly sauté spinach in olive oil with minced garlic.

Brussels sprouts with a balsamic glaze:For a sweet and sour side dish, roast Brussels sprouts until fork-tender and sprinkle with balsamic glaze.

Salad made with cucumber and tomatoes: For a cool side dish, combine thinly sliced cucumbers, cherry tomatoes, red onion, and feta cheese with balsamic dressing.

Wild Rice Pilaf:For a hearty side dish, prepare wild rice with chopped mushrooms, onion, and celery in low-sodium vegetable broth.

Salad made from roasted beets: Beets are roasted until they are soft, after which they are sliced and combined with arugula, goat cheese, and balsamic reduction.

Green beans that have been sautéed: Green beans should be quickly sautéed in olive oil with a sprinkle of almond slivers for crunch.

Cilantro-Lime Quinoa : Adding chopped cilantro, lime juice, and lime zest to cooked quinoa creates a tasty and zesty side dish.

Buttery Corn on the Cob with Chili and Lime: For a hot and tangy side, grill or steam corn on the cob and brush with a mixture of melted butter, chili powder, and lime juice.

Stuffed potatoes with cheddar and broccoli: For a great side dish, bake russet potatoes, remove the meat, combine it with cheddar cheese and broccoli that has been steam-cooked.

Ratatouille, With eggplant, zucchini, bell peppers, tomatoes, and onions cooked in a tomato sauce, make a delectable ratatouille.

Sauteed mushrooms:For a flavorful side dish, sauté sliced mushrooms with garlic, thyme, and a little white wine.

Roasted potatoes with lemon and herbs: For a fragrant and tasty side, roast potato wedges with olive oil, lemon zest, and fresh herbs like rosemary and thyme.

The broad variety of flavors and alternatives in these snack and side dish suggestions can keep your meals interesting while assisting in your weight loss efforts. There is something here to satisfy every preference, whether you're searching for a fast snack or a delectable side.

Chapter 10

Alternative and healthy dessert

Dessert can be a difficult component of a balanced eating plan, especially when trying to lose weight. However, there are lots of dessert options that you can enjoy without feeling bad and strategies to sate your sweet tooth without going off track. We'll look at several delectable dessert substitutes in this part to see how they can keep you on track.

Options for guilt-free desserts

Dessert consumption need not be a sinful indulgence. Here are some dessert options that can satisfy your sweet taste without packing on the sugar or calories:

Fruit Salad:Natural sweetness and a range of vitamins and minerals can be found in a bowl of fresh fruit salad that has been topped with honey and cinnamon.

Greek yogurt parfait (optional): For a creamy and filling treat, layer Greek yogurt with fresh berries, a dash of honey or maple syrup, and a sprinkling of granola or chopped almonds.

Popsicles made from frozen yogurt: For a cool and protein-rich dessert, combine Greek yogurt with your preferred fruit, pour into popsicle molds, and freeze.

Dark Chocolate: Opt for bar chocolate that has at least 70% cacao by weight. Your cravings for chocolate can be sated with a modest piece without eating too much sugar.

Baked apples:Apples are cored, then oats, cinnamon, and a little honey are stuffed within. For a warm and soothing dessert, bake till soft.

Chia Seed Pudding:Chia seeds, almond milk, and a sweetener such agave nectar or vanilla extract are combined to create chia seed pudding. Add fresh fruit to the top for flavor.

Ice cream made with bananas: Ripe bananas are blended till creamy after being frozen. For flavor changes, mix in a small amount of cocoa powder, vanilla essence, or nut butter.

Date and Coconut Rolls: For a naturally sweet treat, combine dates and unsweetened shredded coconut in a food processor, form into bite-sized balls, and chill.

Berry Sorbet:For a cool sorbet, combine frozen mixed berries with a little lemon juice, honey, or agave nectar.

Nut butter-topped rice cakes For a filling and crispy dessert, spread almond or peanut butter on whole-grain rice cakes and top with sliced banana or berries.

Chocolate Avocado Mousse: A creamy chocolate mousse can be made by blending ripe avocados with cocoa powder, a sweetener like honey or maple syrup, and a splash of vanilla extract.

Mini fruit tarts:For a healthier version of fruit tarts, use whole-grain or almond flour for the crust and top with a dollop of Greek yogurt and fresh fruit.

Satisfying Sweet Cravings

These options can aid in satisfying your sweet tooth without jeopardizing your commitment to a healthy lifestyle when you experience strong desires for sweets:

Dried Fruit:A small dose of unsweetened dried fruit, such as raisins or apricots, can offer fiber and natural sweetness.

Frozen Grapes: Frozen grapes have a sorbet-like texture and are a sweet and energizing snack.

Sandwich with Nut Butter and Bananas: Sliced banana and nut butter can be sandwiched between two whole-grain crackers or rice cakes.

Cinnamon Toast:For a warming and delicious snack, top whole-grain toast with a dash of cinnamon and some honey.

Strawberries with a chocolate coating:For a delectable treat, dip fresh strawberries in melted dark chocolate and let them cool.

Trail Mix:For a filling and delicious snack, combine a variety of unsalted nuts, seeds, and a small quantity of dark chocolate chips to make a trail mix.

Baked cinnamon apples:For a warm and fragrant dessert, slice the apples, sprinkle with cinnamon and a little brown sugar or sugar substitute, and bake until soft.

Cinnamon-flavored popcorn:Cinnamon's and a little sprinkling of powdered sugar or a sugar substitute should be added to air-popped popcorn.

Banana Nut Oat Bars: Use mashed bananas, oats, chopped almonds, and a little honey for natural sweetness to make homemade oat bars.

Strawberry-Dipped Yogurt: For a creamy and delicious treat, dip fresh strawberries in Greek yogurt, then freeze until the yogurt sets.

Baked Pears: Cut pears in half, remove the core, and bake the halves until they are cooked. Sprinkle them with cinnamon and drizzle them with honey.

Nutty Energy Balls:In a food processor, combine nuts, seeds, dried fruit, and a little honey or nut butter. Make bite-sized balls out of the mixture for a filling snack.

These dessert substitutes come in a variety of tastes and textures to let you indulge in sweets while still achieving your health and weight loss objectives. Try with different combinations to discover your preferences and produce desserts that satisfy your desires without making you feel bad.

Chapter 11

Meal planning techniques

Maintaining a healthy eating pattern and achieving your weight loss objectives depend on effective meal preparation. The tactics for meal preparation will be covered in this section, including batch cooking, meal freezing, and creating a weekly meal prep schedule.

Batch cooking and meal freezing

You can save time, cut down on food waste, and make sure you always have wholesome options on hand by batch cooking and storing meals. Here's how to maximize this kind of meal preparation:

Select recipes that can be frozen Look for dishes that can be frozen, such as chili, soups, stews, and casseroles. After being frozen and reheated, these foods frequently taste even better.

Spend money on freezer-friendly containers (point b): Purchase a range of freezer-safe containers, including airtight storage containers, freezer bags, and glass containers.

Label and Date:Label each container with the contents and the date of preparation when freezing meals. This guarantees that you use the oldest meals first and makes it simple to recognize what is in the freezer.

Measurement Control: Before freezing, separate large amounts of cooked food into servings for one or two people. Exactly what you need can be quickly thawed and reheated thanks to this.

Cooling Before Freezing: Before putting cooked meals in the freezer, let them cool to room temperature. This stops moisture from building up within the containers and changing the texture of the food.

Freeze in Stages:Rice and pasta should be frozen separately from the sauce or protein when they are part of a meal. When reheated, this avoids overcooking.

Reheat Effectively: Use secure techniques, such as the microwave, stovetop, or oven, depending on the dish, when reheating frozen food. Make sure you heat the food to a safe internal temperature.

Maintain an Inventory: Keep track of the meals you have in your freezer, along with the dates of each meal. This enables you to use leftover food before it degrades.

Rotate Your Stock: To preserve meal freshness and quality, try to use the oldest meals first.

Weekly Meal Preparation Schedule

Making a weekly timetable for meal preparation will speed up the process and guarantee that you always have well-balanced meals on hand. Here's how to establish a productive meal preparation schedule:

Plan your menu for the week by beginning with your a. Choose the recipes you wish to make while considering your dietary objectives and dietary requirements.

Make a Shopping List: Make a thorough shopping list based on the meals you have scheduled. By doing this, you may avoid making impulsive purchases and make sure you have all the materials.

Decide on a prep day and set aside that day of the week as your food preparation day. Sundays are popular, but any day that works for your schedule is OK.

Keep Your Kitchen Organized: Make sure your kitchen is tidy and organized before you start cooking. Make sure you have all the necessary tools and containers and clear the counters.

Focus on preparing ingredients that may be used in several meals, such as cooked proteins, grains, and chopped veggies, while cooking in batches.

Assemble Meals:After preparing the separate ingredients, put together whole meals in containers. Portioning out proteins, grains, and vegetables could be a part of this.

Store Correctly: Make sure to label and store your prepared meals in airtight containers with the date they were made.

Set realistic objectives: Keep in mind how much time you have to prepare meals. Start with a moderate workload and raise it gradually as you get more accustomed to it.

Try New Things and Adapt: Preparing meals is a customized procedure. Try out various menus, ingredients, and tactics until you discover a regimen that suits you the best.

Use Varieties: By mixing up the flavors, cuisines, and ingredients in your weekly meal prep, you can keep your meals interesting.

Be adaptable:Be prepared to alter your meal preparation schedule as necessary because life can be unpredictable. If your prep day is over, locate another time during the week to finish up.

Rejoice in Your Success: Recognize your efforts and the time you've saved during the week. Enjoy a satisfying, wholesome lunch that you prepared for yourself as a reward.

You may make eating healthy more practical and long-lasting by using the meal preparation techniques listed here. It aids in maintaining your weight loss objectives, lessens the temptation to make poor eating choices, and eases the strain brought on by having to prepare meals every day.

Chapter 12

Maintaining motivation

Long-term success in your weight loss journey depends on your ability to stay motivated. In this section, we'll look at methods for keeping your motivation high, such as tracking your progress, recognizing your accomplishments, and overcoming typical obstacles.

Tracking Progress and Rejoicing in Success

Keep a notebook to record your everyday routines, including your eating and exercise. This can aid in pattern recognition, accountability, and little success celebration.

Set Realistic Objectives:Divide your long-term weight loss objective into more manageable, shorter deadlines. Celebrate these accomplishments to show that you are making progress.

Utilize wearable technology and applications to keep track of your exercises, caloric intake, and steps. Goal-setting and progress-tracking tools are also common in many apps.

Take regular shots of your entire body to visibly monitor your development. The ability to see physical improvements in yourself can be a strong incentive.

Measure body metrics as follows: Track changes in your waist, hips, and other body measures using a measuring tape. Changes in measures can occasionally be more obvious than changes in weight.

Honor small-scale victories: Don't only pay attention to the scale's reading. Celebrate accomplishments other than weight loss, such as more energy, better fitness, and better sleep.

Reward Yourself: Reward yourself after reaching a goal. Pick rewards that don't involve food, like a spa day, a new book, or a movie night.

Share Your Progress: Let loved ones know how you're doing with your weight loss. Their support and encouragement may increase your motivation.

Consider joining a support group for weight loss or physical fitness, either in person or online. It might be motivating to discuss struggles and experiences with other people.

Visualize Your Objectives: Make a vision board or imagine your goals in your head. Staying motivated might be aided by visualizing success.

Remind Yourself of Your "Why": Remind yourself frequently of the motivation behind your weight loss efforts. To maintain focus, connect with your inner driving forces.

Chapter 13

Overcoming typical obstacles

Plateaus:Plateaus in weight loss are frequent. Make changes to your diet or workout program if you reach a plateau. To make progress, experiment with various routines or alter your calorie consumption.

Cravings:Cravings can be very strong. To control cravings, have healthier snack options available and engage in mindful eating.

Social Pressure:When it comes to staying on schedule during social occasions, it might be difficult. Prepare ahead by having a healthy snack before the event or bring a dish to share that is also healthy.

Lack of Time: Making time for exercise and meal preparation might be difficult. Set self-care as a priority and look for time-saving methods, such as quick exercises or streamlined food preparation.

Stress:Emotional eating and stress go hand in hand. Find appropriate coping mechanisms for stress, such as yoga, meditation, or counseling.

Lack of motivation: Elements of motivation come and go. Instead than relying exclusively on motivation on days when you lack it, concentrate on consistency and discipline.

Negative inner dialogue: Positive affirmations and self-compassion should be used to replace negative self-talk. Be gentle to yourself, especially when things are difficult.

Overcoming Obstacles: Recognize that obstacles will inevitably arise on the way. Use your mistakes as learning experiences and growth chances.

Seek Professional Assistance: Consider consulting with a certified dietitian or therapist if you struggle to stay motivated or if you have underlying emotional problems with food and weight.

Modify the objectives if necessary: Goals may occasionally need to be modified to fit your current situation and medical requirements. When necessary, don't be scared to modify your goals.

Keep in mind that motivation can change and that obstacles are a natural part of every trip. The most important thing is your capacity to persevere and move forward despite obstacles. You can maintain motivation and accomplish your weight loss objectives with the appropriate techniques and a good outlook.

Conclusion

You should be commended for starting your weight-loss journey and making the decision to give your health and wellbeing priority. Consider the most important tips and techniques you've learned to assist your weight reduction objectives and general health as you get to the end of this guide.

Adopting a Healthier Lifestyle:

You've learned useful information on the fundamentals of a healthier lifestyle throughout this manual, including:

Basics of Nutrition:You now understand how calories, macronutrients, and the value of a balanced diet all relate to weight loss.

Meal preparation:To prepare wholesome and satisfying meals, you have studied meal planning, grocery shopping, and cooking methods.

Food sides and snacks: You've found substitutes to sate your desires and spice up your diet.

Dessert alternatives include: You've looked into guilt-free dessert options so you can indulge in sweets occasionally.

Meal preparation techniques: You've mastered the art of streamlining your meal preparation process through bulk cooking, meal freezing, and weekly plan creation.

Maintaining Motivation: You've learned techniques for maintaining motivation, monitoring your progress, and overcoming typical obstacles.

You can achieve your weight loss objectives as well as improve your general health, have more energy, and feel better by accepting these ideas and incorporating them into your daily life.

Continue Your Weight Loss Journey:

Keep in mind that losing weight is a dynamic process that changes with time. How to continue your journey is as follows:

Maintain the good behaviors you've formed. Consistency is key. Long-term success is built on consistency.

Set new objectives: As you reach your initial weight loss objectives, think about establishing new ones. This might include fitness benchmarks, adjustments to body composition, or other health-related objectives.

Adjust and Change: As your demands change, be willing to make dietary and exercise modifications. As you advance, what initially worked might need to be changed.

Seek Assistance:When faced with difficulties or in need of advice, don't be afraid to ask friends, family, or experts for help.

Continues to engage in mindful eating, which entails being aware of your hunger cues and appreciating each bite. You may be able to keep a positive connection with food as a result.

Take in the View:Keep in mind that adopting a better and more meaningful lifestyle is the goal of your weight loss journey, not just getting there. Enjoy the journey and recognize your accomplishments along the way.

Consider sharing your knowledge and experience with others who might be traveling a similar path. Your advice can encourage and assist others who are trying to improve their health.

In conclusion, it is admirable that you prioritized your health and started a weight-loss journey. You now possess the know-how, the methods, and the resolve needed to make long-lasting, constructive changes in your life thanks to what you have learned from this book. Adopt a healthy lifestyle, keep moving forward with tenacity and resilience, and keep in mind that each step you take will bring you closer to your objectives and a higher standard of living.